PANCREATIC CANCER DIET COOKBOOK FOR BEGINNERS

From Kitchen to Recovery: A Step-by-Step Guide to Crafting Wholesome Meals for Pancreatic Cancer Warrior

McDonnell B. Young

Copyright © 2024 by **McDonnell B. Young**
All rights reserved

No part of this publication may be reproduced, stored in a retrieval system, or transmitted, in any form or by any means, electronic, mechanical, photocopying, recording, or otherwise, without the prior written permission of the author.

The information in this ebook is true and complete to the best of our knowledge. All recommendation are made without guarantee on the part of author or publisher. The author and publisher disclaim any liability in connection with the use of this

Table of Contents

Introduction — 5
    Understanding Pancreatic Cancer — 8
    Role of Diet in Pancreatic Cancer Management — 11
    How to Use This Cookbook — 14

Chapter: 1 Dietary Guidelines for Pancreatic Cancer — 17
    Nutritional Needs and Challenges — 17
    Foods to Include and Avoid — 20
    The Importance of Hydration — 23

Chapter: 2 Breakfast Recipes — 26
    Oatmeal with Blueberries and Almonds — 26
    Smoothie Bowl with Kale, Banana, and Chia Seeds — 28
    Ginger Pear Congee — 30
    Avocado Toast with Poached Egg — 32
    Cottage Cheese with Honey and Walnuts — 34
    Sweet Potato and Lentil Pancakes — 36
    Spiced Pumpkin Porridge — 38
    Scrambled Eggs with Spinach and Mushrooms — 40
    Greek Yoghourt with Mixed Berries and Granola — 42
    Quinoa and Apple Warm Breakfast Salad — 44

Chapter: 3 Lunch Recipes — 46
    Lentil Soup with Carrots and Celery — 46
    Quinoa Salad with Chickpeas and Cucumber — 49

Baked Salmon with Steamed Broccoli	51
Chicken Wraps with Avocado and Spinach	53
Vegetable Stir Fry with Brown Rice	55
Butternut Squash Risotto	58
Tuna Salad with Mixed Greens	60
Turkey and Quinoa Stuffed Peppers	62
Grilled Vegetable and Hummus Flatbread	64
Broccoli and Cauliflower Cheese Bake	66
Chapter: 4 Dinner Recipes	**69**
Grilled Chicken with Quinoa and Roasted Vegetables	69
Baked White Fish with Garlic Spinach	72
Vegetable Lasagna with Ricotta Cheese	74
Stuffed Bell Peppers with Ground Turkey and Herbs	77
Mushroom and Barley Soup	80
Beef Stew with Root Vegetables	82
Roasted Eggplant and Tomato Stew	84
Cod in Parsley Sauce with Mashed Potatoes	86
Sweet Potato Shepherd's Pie	88
Pasta with Pesto and Peas	90
Chapter: 5 Snacks and Sides	**92**
Healthy Snacking Options	92
Recipes for Nutritious Sides	98
Chapter: 6 Beverages and Smoothies	**104**
Juices and Smoothies to Support Hydration and Nutrition	104
Herbal Teas and Their Benefits	108

Chapter: 7 Tips for Eating Well During Treatment 112
    Managing Common Digestive Issues 112
    Meal Planning and Preparation Tips 115
conclusion 118

Introduction

In the quaint town of Willow Creek, Sarah, a nutritionist at the local hospital, noticed a concerning trend among her patients diagnosed with pancreatic cancer. Many struggled not only with their treatment but also with maintaining a healthy diet, which is crucial in managing their symptoms and improving their overall health.

Inspired to make a difference, Sarah decided to create the "Pancreatic Cancer Diet Cookbook for Beginners." She envisioned a guide that would simplify the overwhelming world of nutrition for cancer patients and their families, offering them not just recipes but a beacon of support in their journey.

One sunny morning, Sarah sat down at her old oak desk, armed with medical journals, her clinical experience, and feedback from her patients about their dietary struggles and successes. She meticulously crafted each chapter to address the specific nutritional needs of pancreatic cancer patients, emphasizing foods that were both beneficial and easy to digest.

The cookbook was more than just a collection of recipes; it was a guide infused with compassion and practical advice. Sarah included sections on how to manage common side effects of cancer treatment like nausea and reduced appetite. She provided tips for enhancing flavor for those experiencing taste changes, and her meal plans were designed to be flexible, accommodating the fluctuating energy levels of her readers.

When the "Pancreatic Cancer Diet Cookbook for Beginners" finally hit the shelves of the local bookstore, it wasn't just another cookbook. It was a companion in the kitchens of those battling pancreatic cancer.

Emma, whose father was recently diagnosed with the disease, stumbled upon Sarah's book while searching for resources to help manage his diet. The clear, beginner-friendly explanations and nutritious recipes seemed tailor-made for her father, who had lost his appetite and struggled with the taste alterations caused by his treatment. Emma bought the book immediately, hopeful about the positive changes it promised.

Over the following weeks, Emma noticed a transformation not just in her father's health, but in his spirit. The simple act of preparing a meal from the cookbook became their bonding time. Dishes like the "Ginger Pear Congee" or the "Sweet Potato Shepherd's Pie" were not only palatable and nutritious but also brought a sense of normalcy and joy to their daily lives.

Word of the positive impact of Sarah's cookbook spread quickly throughout Willow Creek and beyond. Testimonials poured in, with families sharing stories of how the recipes brought comfort and nourishment during challenging times. The cookbook became a recommended resource in oncology offices across the county, praised for its thoughtful approach to the dietary needs of cancer patients.

The "Pancreatic Cancer Diet Cookbook for Beginners" ultimately represented more than just food. It was about nurturing hope, fostering well-being, and providing a practical tool for those touched by pancreatic cancer to regain control over an aspect of their lives. For anyone navigating the turbulent waters of such a daunting diagnosis, Sarah's guide offered a much-needed sense of empowerment and reassurance. It wasn't just a good purchase—it was an essential resource that filled kitchens with the aromas of healing and the warmth of care.

Understanding Pancreatic Cancer

Pancreatic cancer begins in the tissues of the pancreas, an essential organ lying behind the lower part of the stomach. This gland plays a crucial role in digestion by producing enzymes that help digest fats, carbohydrates, and proteins. The pancreas also produces insulin and glucagon, hormones that help manage blood sugar. The onset of pancreatic cancer is often insidious, with symptoms that are vague and easily mistaken for less serious conditions, which can delay diagnosis until the cancer is advanced.

When considering dietary needs, pancreatic cancer poses significant challenges due to the pancreas's role in digestion. As the disease progresses, the ability of the pancreas to produce digestive enzymes decreases, leading to problems like weight loss, malnutrition, and steatorrhea (the excretion of abnormal quantities of fat with the feces owing to reduced absorption of fat by the intestine). This makes the nutritional management of patients with pancreatic cancer critical. A diet for individuals with this condition needs to be highly specialized, focusing on maximizing nutrient intake and minimizing digestive distress.

In creating the "Pancreatic Cancer Diet Cookbook for Beginners," there is an emphasis on recipes that are easy to digest and nutrient-rich, suitable for someone with compromised pancreatic function. Foods that are generally soft, well-cooked, and bland can be easier on the stomach, making them ideal for this diet. The inclusion of meals rich in proteins and packed with calories can help combat weight loss and provide the energy that patients critically need.

Another aspect of dietary management is the timing and size of meals. Smaller, more frequent meals can be beneficial for pancreatic cancer patients. Large meals can overwhelm the digestive system, causing discomfort and pain. By providing recipes that are portion-controlled yet nutritious, the cookbook helps patients maintain an adequate intake of food throughout the day.

Furthermore, the cookbook takes into account the common side effects of both the disease and its treatments, such as chemotherapy. Chemotherapy can lead to an increased risk of nausea, vomiting, and taste changes. Therefore, the cookbook includes recipes that incorporate ingredients known to counteract these side effects, like ginger for nausea and recipes that are appealing and flavorful to help with altered taste sensations.

Hydration is another critical factor addressed in the cookbook. Pancreatic cancer patients often struggle with dehydration, especially if experiencing vomiting or diarrhea. The cookbook not only provides recipes for nutritious meals but also includes tips for incorporating fluids throughout the day. This can involve recipes for hydrating foods, suggestions for herbal teas, and easy-to-prepare nutritious smoothies.

Lastly, the cookbook serves as an educational tool for patients and their families, helping them understand why certain foods are chosen and how they benefit the patient. It offers practical advice on how to adjust one's cooking methods and food choices to best support the health of someone facing pancreatic cancer. By integrating these dietary guidelines, the cookbook aims to enhance the quality of life for patients, allowing them to enjoy food in a way that also supports their health and well-being.

Role of Diet in Pancreatic Cancer Management

The role of diet in managing pancreatic cancer is pivotal, as nutrition can significantly impact the effectiveness of treatments and the overall quality of life of patients. Due to the nature of the disease and its treatments, patients often experience digestive difficulties, which can lead to weight loss and malnutrition. A tailored diet, focusing on nutrient-dense foods, can help mitigate these issues by supporting the body's nutritional needs and enhancing the patient's strength and immune function.

Nutritionists emphasize the importance of including easily digestible, high-calorie foods to counteract the weight loss many patients face. Foods high in protein are especially recommended to help repair and build tissue, especially after invasive treatments like surgery or chemotherapy. Including healthy fats from sources like avocados, nuts, and olive oil is also crucial, as these fats provide a dense source of calories and help in the absorption of fat-soluble vitamins which are vital for maintaining body function during treatment.

Hydration plays a critical role in the health of pancreatic cancer patients, especially those undergoing treatment. Adequate fluid intake helps maintain essential bodily functions and can alleviate some side effects of treatments, such as nausea and constipation. The inclusion of hydrating foods, such as fruits and vegetables with high water content, is advised, along with regular fluid intake throughout the day to maintain hydration.

Certain foods and cooking methods are more suitable for managing symptoms common in pancreatic cancer patients, such as nausea and a sensitive stomach. For instance, ginger is renowned for its ability to alleviate nausea and is a versatile ingredient that can be included in various recipes within the cookbook. Additionally, preparing foods that are baked or steamed rather than fried can help prevent aggravating digestive issues, making meals more tolerable and appealing to patients.

The timing and size of meals can also significantly affect how well pancreatic cancer patients can manage their diet and maintain their intake of necessary nutrients. Eating small, frequent meals rather than three large ones can help maximize nutrient intake when appetite is low and digestion is compromised. This approach also helps stabilize blood sugar levels, which is crucial since pancreatic cancer can impact insulin production and exacerbate or lead to diabetes.

For those undergoing chemotherapy and radiation, there are additional dietary considerations to take into account. These treatments can alter taste perceptions, making previously enjoyable foods seem unpalatable. Experimenting with seasonings and flavors can help in rediscovering pleasure in eating. The cookbook provides recipes that are not only nutritious but also focus on a variety of flavors and textures to cater to changing tastes and preferences, making meals more enjoyable and diverse.

Overall, managing diet in pancreatic cancer is a dynamic process, requiring adjustments based on treatment phases and individual responses. The cookbook serves as a guide to navigate these complexities, offering recipes that address common dietary challenges faced by patients. It stands as a valuable tool for patients and caregivers alike, aiming to ease the burden of diet management and improve the effectiveness of overall treatment and care. Through proper nutrition, patients can see improved treatment outcomes, better quality of life, and potentially, a more favorable prognosis.

How to Use This Cookbook

When embarking on the journey through the "Pancreatic Cancer Diet Cookbook for Beginners," it's essential to consider the unique dietary needs that accompany the treatment of pancreatic cancer. The recipes within this book are specifically designed to be gentle on the stomach, easy to digest, and nutritious, providing the body with the necessary strength to combat the illness and endure treatment side effects. Each recipe includes detailed nutritional information to help you track the intake of key nutrients vital for maintaining energy levels and overall health during this challenging time.

Understanding the physical challenges faced by many patients, such as decreased appetite and altered taste sensations, this cookbook offers a variety of flavors and textures to cater to shifting preferences. The meals are structured to be appealing and satisfying, even when your appetite might be waning. Tips for enhancing or modifying flavors to suit your current taste capabilities are provided, ensuring that every meal not only nourishes but also pleases the palate.

The cookbook is also designed to accommodate the varying levels of energy cancer patients experience. Recipes are categorized by their preparation time and effort required, allowing you to choose suitable meals for days when energy is low. Quick, simple dishes that require minimal standing or preparation time are highlighted, making it easier to continue eating well even on your toughest days.

Adaptability is a key feature of this guide, acknowledging that dietary needs can change over the course of treatment. Suggestions for substitutions are provided for ingredients that might not always be available or appealing, ensuring that meals can be tailored to personal tastes and nutritional requirements. This flexibility makes it possible to maintain a balanced diet that supports healing and health.

The book encourages involvement from family and friends, recognizing that cooking and meal preparation can be a communal activity that offers emotional support and practical help. The recipes are designed to be prepared by anyone, regardless of their cooking skill level, which makes it easier for caregivers to get involved in the dietary care of their loved ones.

In addition to the recipes, the book serves as an educational tool, equipping readers with knowledge about how different foods and nutrients can affect the body during pancreatic cancer treatment. It explains the reasoning behind the inclusion of certain foods and the exclusion of others, empowering you with the understanding needed to make informed decisions about your diet.

Lastly, the cookbook is a resource for continuous learning and adaptation. It invites feedback and suggests keeping a food diary to monitor how certain foods affect your body and spirit. This ongoing engagement with both the meals and the body's response helps fine-tune dietary choices, ensuring they remain aligned with the body's needs as circumstances evolve. The "Pancreatic Cancer Diet Cookbook for Beginners" is more than just a collection of recipes—it's a companion in your journey to health, tailored to help navigate the complexities of dietary management in pancreatic cancer with ease and confidence.

Chapter: 1 Dietary Guidelines for Pancreatic Cancer

Nutritional Needs and Challenges

Patients diagnosed with pancreatic cancer face unique nutritional needs and challenges that are critical to consider in order to maintain body weight and strength during treatment. The disease itself, along with the effects of chemotherapy and radiation, can significantly impact digestion and absorption of nutrients. Weight loss and malnutrition are common, as the pancreas plays a crucial role in breaking down fats, proteins, and carbohydrates. Therefore, meals designed for these patients often focus on high caloric intake and easy digestibility to combat these issues.

The altered function of the pancreas often leads to enzyme insufficiency, which makes it difficult for the body to absorb fat properly. This results in steatorrhea, where fat is excreted undigested, and can lead to significant weight loss and malnutrition. To address this, patients are typically advised to include enzyme supplements with their meals to aid digestion. Recipes in the cookbook incorporate easily digestible fats and are paired with guidance on how and when to take enzyme replacements to optimize nutrient absorption.

Protein needs are also heightened in pancreatic cancer patients to help repair and build tissue, especially if they are undergoing surgery or other forms of aggressive therapy. Including adequate protein is essential to help maintain muscle mass and strength, which can be adversely affected during treatment. The cookbook provides recipes rich in lean proteins that are tender and easy to chew, which helps in cases where patients may also be experiencing nausea or a sore mouth from treatment.

Carbohydrate intake is equally important, though it should be carefully managed because many patients experience fluctuations in blood sugar levels due to the cancer's impact on insulin production. The recipes include complex carbohydrates that provide a slower release of energy, helping to maintain stable blood sugar, and detailed notes on how to adjust these for those closely monitoring their glycemic control.

Hydration is another crucial aspect covered in the cookbook. Pancreatic cancer patients can experience dehydration due to vomiting or diarrhea. The cookbook encourages the intake of fluids through not just beverages but also through soups, broths, and foods high in water content. There are also tips on recognizing signs of dehydration and how to effectively address it within a dietary context.

Vitamins and minerals deficiencies are common due to malabsorption, and replenishing these is crucial for maintaining the body's defenses against infection and supporting overall health. The cookbook emphasizes foods rich in essential vitamins and minerals, such as fruits, vegetables, and fortified foods, and includes advice on when supplementation might be necessary under a healthcare provider's guidance.

Lastly, managing dietary fat is particularly challenging but crucial. While high-fat foods can exacerbate digestive issues, some fat is necessary for energy and to aid in the absorption of fat-soluble vitamins. The cookbook offers recipes that balance the need for fats with the common digestive capabilities of pancreatic cancer patients, providing options for healthy fats like avocado and nuts that are more easily tolerated. The comprehensive approach in the cookbook ensures that patients not only receive the nutrients needed to support their treatment and recovery but also enjoy a quality of life through better managed dietary habits.

Foods to Include and Avoid

Navigating the dietary landscape when managing pancreatic cancer involves understanding which foods can support health and which may exacerbate symptoms. Foods rich in antioxidants, such as fruits and vegetables, are encouraged due to their ability to combat oxidative stress and reduce inflammation. Brightly colored vegetables and fruits, like berries, carrots, and leafy greens, provide essential vitamins and minerals that can help bolster the immune system, which is crucial during cancer treatment.

Whole grains are another group of foods that play a beneficial role in the diet of pancreatic cancer patients. These grains, including oats, barley, and quinoa, are high in fiber, which helps maintain bowel health. Many patients undergoing cancer treatment may experience digestive issues, and incorporating fiber-rich foods can aid digestion and prevent constipation. It's important, however, to increase fiber intake gradually to assess tolerance, as some individuals might experience bloating or gas.

Lean proteins are essential for healing and repair of tissues, and maintaining muscle mass in pancreatic cancer patients. Options like chicken, turkey, fish, and legumes not only provide vital protein but are also generally easier to digest compared to red meats. Fish, particularly those rich in omega-3 fatty acids like salmon and mackerel, can be especially beneficial due to their anti-inflammatory properties, which might help reduce side effects associated with cancer treatments.

Healthy fats are critical in a pancreatic cancer diet as they help absorb fat-soluble vitamins and provide a dense source of energy, which is significant for patients who may struggle with weight loss due to decreased appetite. Sources of healthy fats include avocados, nuts, seeds, and olive oil. These fats should be consumed in moderation, and the preparation methods should be gentle, favoring baking or steaming over frying to avoid digestive discomfort.

Conversely, there are certain foods that should be limited or avoided. Foods high in simple sugars and refined carbohydrates can cause rapid spikes in blood sugar and energy levels, leading to crashes that can exacerbate fatigue and impair immune function. Sweets, white bread, and processed foods fall into this category and should be consumed sparingly, if at all, to avoid complicating the body's energy regulation.

Fried and fatty foods are particularly hard on the pancreas and can aggravate digestive symptoms, making them less ideal for those with pancreatic cancer. High-fat meats, deep-fried foods, and rich, creamy sauces can increase the workload on the digestive system and should be avoided to prevent nausea and digestive upset. Instead, cooking methods that require less oil and fat, such as grilling or steaming, are recommended.

Lastly, alcohol and caffeine can also pose problems for pancreatic cancer patients. Alcohol can be hard on the liver and pancreas, potentially worsening symptoms and impacting treatment outcomes. Caffeine can interfere with sleep and may irritate the digestive system. Limiting or avoiding these beverages can help manage symptoms more effectively, allowing for a smoother treatment process and better overall health management during this challenging time.

The Importance of Hydration

Hydration is paramount for individuals battling pancreatic cancer, as the body requires adequate fluids to function optimally and handle the stresses of cancer and its treatment. Water plays a critical role in every cellular activity, from aiding digestion to ensuring nutrients are effectively transported throughout the body. It also helps manage the side effects of medication and can alleviate symptoms such as nausea, which are common during cancer treatments.

Patients with pancreatic cancer often face challenges with hydration due to symptoms like vomiting or diarrhea, which can lead to dehydration quickly if not monitored closely. Dehydration can exacerbate fatigue, reduce the effectiveness of medications, and make side effects more severe. Therefore, maintaining fluid intake isn't just about quenching thirst; it's a crucial component of the overall treatment plan to keep the body resilient against the aggressiveness of both the disease and the treatment.

The cookbook provides practical tips for increasing fluid intake, even when the desire to drink might be diminished. Including a variety of hydrating foods in the diet, such as fruits and vegetables with high water content, soups, and broths, is an effective way to supplement direct fluid intake. These options provide hydration while also offering nutritional benefits, which is a dual advantage for patients whose appetite might be waning.

Beyond just water, the guide discusses the importance of balancing electrolytes which are vital for regulating body functions. Cancer treatments can disrupt mineral balances, making it necessary to include sources of electrolytes like sodium, potassium, and magnesium in the diet. Coconut water, sports drinks designed for medical use, and electrolyte-enhanced waters are options detailed in the cookbook, each providing different benefits to suit individual needs and preferences.

For patients experiencing a sore mouth or throat, a common side effect of some cancer therapies, the cookbook suggests hydration solutions that are soothing and gentle. Warm herbal teas, which are both calming and hydrating, can provide relief while ensuring fluid intake is maintained. The inclusion of options like gelatin desserts and pudding can also serve the dual purpose of hydration and energy provision through calories.

The book also addresses the need to monitor fluid intake and output carefully, with advice on recognizing signs of dehydration early. This proactive approach is essential as dehydration can progress quickly and become severe, leading to further complications. Caregivers are also provided with guidelines to help them support the patient in maintaining adequate hydration.

In sum, the cookbook emphasizes that while nutrition is vitally important for pancreatic cancer patients, hydration is equally critical. The strategies provided are designed to integrate easily into daily routines, ensuring that maintaining hydration is not a burden but a seamlessly managed component of the overall care plan. Through its comprehensive approach, the cookbook equips patients and their caregivers with the knowledge and tools necessary to tackle one of the fundamental challenges in cancer care—staying adequately hydrated.

Chapter: 2 Breakfast Recipes

Oatmeal with Blueberries and Almonds

Ingredients:

- 1 cup of rolled oats
- 2 cups of water or milk for creamier texture
- 1/2 cup fresh blueberries
- 1/4 cup slivered almonds
- 1 tablespoon of honey or maple syrup (optional)
- 1/4 teaspoon of cinnamon (optional)

Instructions:

1. In a small saucepan, bring the water or milk to a boil. Add the rolled oats and simmer on low heat, stirring occasionally, until the oats are soft and have absorbed most of the liquid, about 5-7 minutes.
2. Remove the pan from heat and stir in the blueberries, almonds, and optional honey and cinnamon. Let the oatmeal sit for a minute or two for the flavors to meld.
3. Serve warm, adding extra milk or water if a thinner consistency is preferred.

Nutritional Information (per serving):

- Calories: 310
- Protein: 9 grams
- Fat: 9 grams (1 gram saturated, the rest unsaturated)
- Carbohydrates: 50 grams
- Fiber: 7 grams
- Sugar: 10 grams (excluding optional honey or syrup)

Serving Size:

- Makes 2 servings

Cooking Time:

- Total preparation and cooking time: Approximately 10-12 minutes

Smoothie Bowl with Kale, Banana, and Chia Seeds

Ingredients:
- 1 cup chopped kale, stems removed
- 1 ripe banana
- 2 tablespoons chia seeds
- 1/2 cup unsweetened almond milk (or any preferred milk)
- 1/4 cup plain Greek yogurt
- 1 tablespoon honey (optional, for added sweetness)
- 1/2 cup assorted fresh berries (for topping)
- A sprinkle of unsweetened coconut flakes (for topping)

Instructions:
1. In a blender, combine the kale, banana, almond milk, Greek yogurt, and honey. Blend until smooth.
2. Pour the smoothie mixture into a bowl.
3. Sprinkle the chia seeds evenly over the smoothie.
4. Garnish with fresh berries and coconut flakes.
5. Serve immediately.

Nutritional Information:
- Calories: 340
- Protein: 8 g
- Fat: 10 g (Saturated Fat: 1 g)

- Carbohydrates: 55 g (Fibers: 12 g, Sugars: 20 g)
- Sodium: 85 mg

Serving Size: 1 bowl

Cooking Time: 10 minutes (prep and assembly)

Ginger Pear Congee

Ingredients for Ginger Pear Congee:

- 1 cup jasmine rice, rinsed
- 4 cups water
- 1 cup unsweetened almond milk
- 1 fresh pear, peeled and diced
- 2 teaspoons freshly grated ginger
- 1 tablespoon honey (optional, depending on dietary needs)
- Pinch of salt

Instructions:

1. Combine the rinsed jasmine rice and water in a large pot. Bring to a boil.
2. Reduce the heat to a low simmer, cover, and cook for about 20 minutes, occasionally stirring, until the rice is soft and begins to break down.
3. Add the almond milk, diced pear, and grated ginger to the pot. Stir well to incorporate.
4. Continue to simmer for an additional 10 minutes, or until the congee is creamy and the pear pieces are tender.
5. Stir in honey if desired and a pinch of salt for taste.
6. Serve warm, adding extra almond milk if a thinner consistency is preferred.

Nutritional Information:

Each serving of Ginger Pear Congee offers a gentle balance of carbohydrates and fiber, with the ginger providing anti-inflammatory benefits and the pear offering a good source of vitamin C and fiber. The almond milk adds a touch of protein and is typically fortified with calcium and vitamin D.

Serving Size:

This recipe serves four, making it ideal for individual servings or small families.

Cooking Time:

Preparation and cooking for the Ginger Pear Congee take approximately 40 minutes, making it a feasible option for a nourishing, easy-to-digest breakfast.

Avocado Toast with Poached Egg

Ingredients:

- 1 ripe avocado
- 2 eggs
- 2 slices of whole-grain bread
- 1 teaspoon of lemon juice
- Salt and pepper to taste
- Optional garnishes: Chopped cilantro, cherry tomatoes, or a sprinkle of flaxseed

Instructions:

1. Begin by poaching the eggs. Bring a pot of water to a light simmer. Add a small splash of vinegar. Crack each egg into a small cup or bowl and gently pour them one at a time into the simmering water. Let them cook for 3 to 4 minutes, depending on how runny you prefer your yolk. Remove with a slotted spoon and set aside.
2. While the eggs are poaching, toast the bread slices to your desired crispiness.
3. Peel and pit the avocado. In a bowl, mash the avocado with the lemon juice, salt, and pepper.
4. Spread the mashed avocado evenly onto the toasted bread slices.
5. Place a poached egg on each slice of avocado toast.

6. Add optional garnishes like chopped cilantro, cherry tomatoes, or a sprinkle of flaxseed to enhance the flavor and nutritional value.

Nutritional Information (per serving):

- Calories: 290
- Protein: 12 g
- Fat: 20 g (healthy fats from avocado)
- Carbohydrates: 20 g
- Fiber: 7 g
- Sodium: 200 mg

Serving Size:

This recipe serves 1 person. Each serving includes two pieces of avocado toast, each topped with a poached egg.

Cooking Time:

The total cooking time is approximately 15 minutes. This includes the time to poach the eggs and prepare the avocado spread, ensuring a quick yet nutritious meal suitable for a morning routine.

Cottage Cheese with Honey and Walnuts

Ingredients:

- 1 cup low-fat cottage cheese
- 2 tablespoons honey
- 1/4 cup walnuts, chopped
- Optional: a pinch of cinnamon or sliced fresh fruits for topping

Instructions:

1. Place the cottage cheese in a serving bowl.
2. Drizzle honey over the cottage cheese.
3. Sprinkle chopped walnuts on top.
4. If desired, add a pinch of cinnamon or top with fresh fruit slices for added flavor and nutrition.
5. Serve immediately or chill in the refrigerator for 30 minutes if a cooler breakfast is preferred.

Nutritional Information (per serving):

- Calories: 350
- Protein: 19 g
- Fat: 17 g (with only 3 g of saturated fat)
- Carbohydrates: 27 g

- Fiber: 2 g
- Sodium: 500 mg

Serving Size:
- This recipe serves 1 person.

Cooking Time:
- Preparation takes about 5 minutes, with no cooking required.

Sweet Potato and Lentil Pancakes

Ingredients:

- 1 cup cooked and mashed sweet potato
- 1/2 cup pureed cooked red lentils
- 2 large eggs
- 1/4 cup whole wheat flour
- 1/2 teaspoon baking powder
- 1/4 teaspoon salt
- 1/2 teaspoon ground cinnamon
- 1/4 teaspoon nutmeg
- Olive oil or coconut oil for cooking

Instructions:

1. In a large mixing bowl, combine the mashed sweet potato and pureed lentils.
2. Beat in the eggs until the mixture is well combined.
3. Add the whole wheat flour, baking powder, salt, cinnamon, and nutmeg to the sweet potato mixture. Stir until just combined; the batter should be thick.
4. Heat a non-stick skillet over medium heat and brush with a small amount of oil.
5. Pour 1/4 cup of batter for each pancake onto the hot skillet. Cook for 2-3 minutes on each side or until the pancakes are golden brown and cooked through.

6. Serve warm with a drizzle of honey or a dollop of Greek yogurt if desired.

Nutritional Information per serving:

- Calories: 150
- Protein: 6 grams
- Carbohydrates: 23 grams
- Dietary Fiber: 4 grams
- Sugars: 3 grams
- Fat: 4 grams

Serving Size:

- Makes about 8 pancakes; serving size is 2 pancakes.

Cooking Time:

- Prep Time: 15 minutes
- Cook Time: 15 minutes
- Total Time: 30 minutes

Spiced Pumpkin Porridge

Ingredients:

- 1/2 cup rolled oats
- 1 cup almond milk or water
- 1/2 cup pureed pumpkin (canned or fresh)
- 1/4 teaspoon ground cinnamon
- 1/8 teaspoon ground nutmeg
- 1/8 teaspoon ground ginger
- 1 tablespoon maple syrup or honey (optional)
- 1 tablespoon flaxseed, ground (for added fiber and omega-3 fatty acids)

Instructions:

1. In a small saucepan, combine the oats and almond milk or water. Bring to a boil over medium heat.
2. Reduce the heat to low and stir in the pumpkin puree. Simmer, stirring frequently, until the oats are soft and the mixture has thickened, about 5 to 7 minutes.
3. Remove from heat and stir in the cinnamon, nutmeg, ginger, and maple syrup or honey if using.
4. Let the porridge sit for a couple of minutes to thicken further and then serve warm.
5. Sprinkle ground flaxseed on top just before serving for an extra nutritional boost.

Nutritional Information:

Each serving of this porridge offers a balanced mix of carbohydrates, fiber, and protein, along with a healthy dose of vitamins like vitamin A from the pumpkin, which is important for immune function and skin health. The spices not only enhance flavor but also provide anti-inflammatory benefits, which can be helpful in managing inflammation associated with cancer and its treatment.

Serving Size:

This recipe serves one but can easily be doubled or tripled to accommodate more people or to prepare additional servings for later.

Cooking Time:

Total preparation and cooking time is approximately 10-15 minutes, making it a quick and easy option for mornings when time or energy might be limited.

Scrambled Eggs with Spinach and Mushrooms

Ingredients:

- 2 large eggs
- 1/2 cup fresh spinach, chopped
- 1/4 cup mushrooms, sliced
- 1 tablespoon olive oil
- Salt and pepper to taste
- 1 tablespoon low-fat milk (optional, for creamier eggs)

Instructions:

1. Heat the olive oil in a non-stick skillet over medium heat.
2. Add the sliced mushrooms to the skillet and sauté until they begin to soften, about 3-5 minutes.
3. Add the chopped spinach to the skillet and cook until the spinach wilts, about 1-2 minutes.
4. In a bowl, whisk the eggs with milk (if using), salt, and pepper.
5. Pour the egg mixture into the skillet over the sautéed mushrooms and spinach.
6. Stir gently with a spatula, allowing the eggs to cook slowly and scramble. Cook to the desired firmness.
7. Serve warm.

Nutritional Information:

- Calories: 215
- Protein: 13 g
- Fat: 16 g
- Carbohydrates: 3 g
- Fiber: 1 g
- Sugar: 1 g

Serving Size:

- This recipe serves 1, providing a substantial, nutrient-dense start to the day without being overly filling, which is crucial for patients who may experience decreased appetite.

Cooking Time:

- Total preparation and cooking time is approximately 15 minutes, making it a quick and efficient option for a nourishing breakfast.

Greek Yoghourt with Mixed Berries and Granola

Ingredients:
- 1 cup Greek yogurt (plain, unsweetened)
- 1/2 cup mixed berries (blueberries, raspberries, strawberries)
- 1/4 cup granola (preferably low in sugar and high in fiber)
- 1 tablespoon honey or maple syrup (optional, for sweetness)

Instructions:
1. In a serving bowl, place the Greek yogurt.
2. Top the yogurt with the mixed berries.
3. Sprinkle granola over the berries.
4. Drizzle honey or maple syrup over the top if a sweeter taste is desired.
5. Serve immediately to enjoy the crunch of the granola.

Nutritional Information:
- Calories: 310 kcal
- Protein: 20 g
- Carbohydrates: 35 g
- Fat: 10 g
- Fiber: 4 g
- Sugar: 20 g (includes natural sugars from the berries and any added sweeteners)

Serving Size:

- This recipe serves 1. It can be scaled up to serve more, keeping the proportions the same to ensure each serving contains the right balance of nutrients.

Cooking Time:

- Preparation time: 5 minutes
- No cooking required

Quinoa and Apple Warm Breakfast Salad

Ingredients:

- 1 cup quinoa, rinsed
- 2 cups water
- 2 medium apples, diced
- 1 teaspoon cinnamon
- 1 tablespoon honey
- 1/4 cup chopped walnuts
- 1/4 cup dried cranberries

Instructions:

1. In a medium saucepan, bring the 2 cups of water to a boil. Add the rinsed quinoa and reduce the heat to a simmer. Cover and cook for 15 minutes, or until the water is absorbed and the quinoa is tender.
2. While the quinoa is cooking, dice the apples and set aside.
3. Once the quinoa is cooked, fluff it with a fork and mix in the diced apples, cinnamon, honey, chopped walnuts, and dried cranberries.
4. Stir the mixture over low heat just until everything is warm, about 2-3 minutes.
5. Serve warm, perhaps with a dollop of yogurt or a drizzle of additional honey if desired.

Nutritional Information:

- Calories: 235 per serving
- Protein: 6 grams
- Fat: 5 grams
- Carbohydrates: 42 grams
- Fiber: 5 grams
- Sugar: 15 grams

Serving Size: Makes 4 servings

Cooking Time: 20 minutes

Chapter: 3 Lunch Recipes

Lentil Soup with Carrots and Celery

Ingredients:

- 1 cup dried lentils, rinsed
- 4 cups low-sodium vegetable broth
- 1 medium onion, diced
- 2 carrots, peeled and diced
- 2 stalks celery, diced
- 2 cloves garlic, minced
- 1 teaspoon ground cumin
- 1/2 teaspoon dried thyme
- Salt and pepper, to taste
- Optional: chopped parsley for garnish

Instructions:

1. In a large pot, heat a splash of water over medium heat. Add the onion, carrots, and celery, and cook until they are softened, about 5 minutes.
2. Stir in the garlic, cumin, and thyme, and cook for an additional 1 minute until fragrant.
3. Add the rinsed lentils and vegetable broth. Bring the mixture to a boil, then reduce the heat to low, cover, and simmer for about 25-30 minutes, or until the lentils are tender.

4. Season with salt and pepper to taste. Serve hot, garnished with chopped parsley if desired.

Nutritional Information:
Each serving of this soup provides a balanced mix of nutrients beneficial for pancreatic cancer patients, including:
- Calories: Approximately 180
- Protein: 12 grams
- Fat: Less than 1 gram
- Carbohydrates: 30 grams
- Fiber: 15 grams
- Sodium: Varies depending on the use of salt and type of vegetable broth

Serving Size:
This recipe yields about 4 servings, making it easy to prepare in advance and store for several days, ensuring a ready-to-eat option that simplifies meal planning.

Cooking Time:
The total preparation and cooking time for the Lentil Soup with Carrots and Celery is approximately 40 minutes, which includes the initial sautéing of vegetables and the simmering time to cook the lentils thoroughly. This quick and straightforward preparation ensures that valuable nutrients are preserved and the

flavors meld beautifully, offering a soothing and satisfying meal that is both therapeutic and delightful.

Quinoa Salad with Chickpeas and Cucumber

Ingredients:

- 1 cup quinoa
- 2 cups water
- 1 cup canned chickpeas, rinsed and drained
- 1 large cucumber, diced
- 1 small red onion, finely chopped
- 1 red bell pepper, diced
- 1/4 cup fresh parsley, chopped
- 2 tablespoons olive oil
- Juice of 1 lemon
- Salt and pepper to taste

Instructions:

1. Rinse the quinoa under cold running water until the water runs clear. Combine the rinsed quinoa and water in a medium saucepan. Bring to a boil, then cover and reduce to a simmer for 15 minutes, or until the water is absorbed and the quinoa is tender.
2. Fluff the cooked quinoa with a fork and allow it to cool to room temperature.
3. In a large mixing bowl, combine the cooled quinoa, chickpeas, cucumber, red onion, and red bell pepper.

4. In a small bowl, whisk together the olive oil, lemon juice, salt, and pepper. Pour this dressing over the quinoa mixture and toss to coat evenly.

5. Gently stir in the chopped parsley just before serving.

Nutritional Information:

- Calories: 210 per serving
- Protein: 6 grams
- Fat: 7 grams (1 gram saturated)
- Carbohydrates: 33 grams
- Fiber: 5 grams
- Sodium: 200 mg

Serving Size:

- This recipe serves 4. Each serving is approximately 1 cup.

Cooking Time:

- Total preparation and cooking time is about 30 minutes.

Baked Salmon with Steamed Broccoli

Ingredients:

- 4 salmon fillets (6 ounces each)
- 2 tablespoons olive oil
- 1 teaspoon garlic powder
- Salt and pepper to taste
- 1 lemon, sliced into rounds
- 4 cups of broccoli florets
- 1 tablespoon of water

Instructions:

1. Preheat your oven to 400 degrees Fahrenheit (200 degrees Celsius).
2. Line a baking sheet with parchment paper and place the salmon fillets on the sheet, skin side down.
3. Drizzle olive oil over the salmon. Sprinkle with garlic powder, salt, and pepper. Top each fillet with two lemon slices.
4. In a separate oven-proof dish, toss the broccoli florets with the remaining olive oil, salt, and a tablespoon of water. Cover the dish with aluminum foil.
5. Place both the salmon and broccoli in the oven. Bake the salmon for 12-15 minutes or until it flakes easily with a fork. Steam the broccoli in the oven alongside the salmon for about 10-12 minutes, until tender but still crisp.

6. Serve the salmon and broccoli hot, with additional lemon wedges on the side for squeezing.

Nutritional Information:

Each serving of this meal provides approximately:
- Calories: 345
- Protein: 34g
- Fat: 20g (saturated fat: 3g)
- Carbohydrates: 10g
- Fiber: 4g
- Sodium: 75mg

Serving Size:

This recipe serves 4, with each serving consisting of one salmon fillet and a cup of steamed broccoli.

Cooking Time:

Preparation time is about 10 minutes, and cooking time is approximately 15 minutes, making for a total of about 25 minutes from start to finish.

Chicken Wraps with Avocado and Spinach

Ingredients:

- 2 whole wheat tortillas
- 1 cooked chicken breast, thinly sliced
- 1 ripe avocado, peeled and sliced
- 1 cup fresh spinach leaves
- 1/2 small red onion, thinly sliced
- 2 tablespoons Greek yogurt
- 1 tablespoon olive oil
- 1 teaspoon lemon juice
- Salt and pepper to taste

Instructions:

1. In a small bowl, mix the Greek yogurt, olive oil, lemon juice, salt, and pepper to create a dressing.
2. Lay out the whole wheat tortillas on a clean surface.
3. Spread the dressing evenly over each tortilla.
4. Arrange the chicken slices down the center of each tortilla.
5. Top the chicken with avocado slices, spinach, and red onion.
6. Carefully roll the tortillas tightly around the filling to form the wraps.
7. Cut each wrap in half diagonally and serve immediately.

Nutritional Information:

Each serving (1 wrap) typically provides approximately:

- Calories: 400
- Protein: 28 grams
- Fat: 20 grams (with a focus on monounsaturated fats from the avocado)
- Carbohydrates: 33 grams
- Fiber: 6 grams
- Sodium: 200 mg

Serving Size:

This recipe serves 2, with each person getting one full wrap.

Cooking Time:

Preparation time is around 10 minutes, with no additional cooking required if using pre-cooked chicken breast. This makes it a quick and convenient option for a nourishing lunch that doesn't require much time or energy to prepare.

Vegetable Stir Fry with Brown Rice

Ingredients:

- 1 cup brown rice
- 2 cups water
- 1 tablespoon olive oil
- 1 small onion, thinly sliced
- 2 cloves garlic, minced
- 1 bell pepper, julienned
- 1 zucchini, sliced
- 1 carrot, julienned
- 1 cup broccoli florets
- 2 tablespoons low-sodium soy sauce
- 1 tablespoon ginger, freshly grated
- 1 teaspoon sesame oil
- Optional: 1 tablespoon sesame seeds for garnish

Instructions:

1. Start by cooking the brown rice. In a medium saucepan, bring 2 cups of water to a boil. Add the brown rice, reduce the heat to low, cover, and simmer for about 45 minutes, or until the water is absorbed and the rice is tender.
2. While the rice cooks, heat the olive oil in a large skillet or wok over medium-high heat. Add the onion and garlic, sautéing until the onion becomes translucent.

3. Add the bell pepper, zucchini, carrot, and broccoli to the skillet. Stir fry for about 5-7 minutes, or until the vegetables are just tender but still crisp.

4. Stir in the soy sauce and ginger, mixing thoroughly to ensure the vegetables are well-coated.

5. Reduce the heat to low, and drizzle the sesame oil over the vegetables, tossing gently to combine.

6. Serve the stir-fried vegetables over the cooked brown rice. Garnish with sesame seeds if desired.

Nutritional Information:

- Calories: 235 per serving
- Protein: 6 g
- Carbohydrates: 44 g
- Fat: 5 g
- Fiber: 5 g
- Sodium: 300 mg

Serving Size:

This recipe serves 4, with each serving consisting of about 1/2 cup of cooked rice and 1 cup of stir-fried vegetables.

Cooking Time:

Preparation time is approximately 15 minutes, and cooking time is around 60 minutes, including the time to cook the rice.

Butternut Squash Risotto

Ingredients for Butternut Squash Risotto:

- 1 medium butternut squash (peeled, seeded, and cubed)
- 1 tablespoon olive oil
- 4 cups low-sodium chicken or vegetable broth
- 1 small onion, finely chopped
- 1 cup Arborio rice
- 1/2 cup dry white wine (optional; substitute with broth if avoiding alcohol)
- 1/4 cup grated Parmesan cheese
- Salt and pepper to taste
- Fresh sage leaves for garnish

Instructions:

1. Preheat the oven to 400°F (200°C). Toss the butternut squash cubes with olive oil and spread them on a baking sheet. Roast for 25-30 minutes, or until tender and lightly browned.
2. In a saucepan, warm the broth over medium heat.
3. In another saucepan, sauté the onion in a little olive oil until translucent. Add the Arborio rice and stir for about 2 minutes.
4. Add the white wine to the rice and onion mixture, and cook until the liquid is nearly absorbed.

5. Begin adding the warm broth to the rice one ladle at a time, stirring constantly and allowing each ladle of broth to be absorbed before adding the next.

6. When the rice is creamy and just tender (about 20 minutes), stir in the roasted butternut squash.

7. Remove from heat and stir in Parmesan cheese. Season with salt and pepper to taste, and garnish with fresh sage leaves before serving.

Nutritional Information per serving:

- Calories: 280
- Protein: 6g
- Carbohydrates: 53g
- Fat: 5g
- Fiber: 3g
- Sodium: 150mg

Serving Size:

This recipe serves 4 people.

Cooking Time:

Total preparation and cooking time is approximately 55 minutes.

Tuna Salad with Mixed Greens

Ingredients:

- 1 can (5 ounces) of tuna in water, drained
- 2 cups mixed salad greens (spinach, arugula, and romaine)
- 1/4 cup sliced cucumbers
- 1/4 cup cherry tomatoes, halved
- 1/4 cup shredded carrots
- 2 tablespoons olive oil
- 1 tablespoon lemon juice
- Salt and pepper to taste
- Optional: 1 tablespoon of chopped fresh herbs (such as dill or parsley)

Instructions:

1. In a large salad bowl, combine the mixed greens, sliced cucumbers, cherry tomatoes, and shredded carrots.
2. In a small bowl, flake the drained tuna with a fork and add it to the salad mixture.
3. In a separate small bowl, whisk together olive oil, lemon juice, salt, and pepper to create a dressing.
4. Pour the dressing over the salad and toss gently to coat all the ingredients evenly.
5. If using, sprinkle the chopped herbs over the top for added flavor.
6. Serve immediately to ensure the greens stay crisp.

Nutritional Information:

- Calories: 310
- Protein: 25g
- Carbohydrates: 8g
- Fat: 21g (Saturated Fat: 3g; Monounsaturated Fat: 12g)
- Fiber: 3g
- Sodium: 390mg

Serving Size:

- This recipe serves 1 person as a full meal or 2 people as a side salad.

Cooking Time:

- Preparation time: 10 minutes
- No cooking required

Turkey and Quinoa Stuffed Peppers

Ingredients:
- 4 large bell peppers, any color, tops cut away and seeds removed
- 1 tablespoon olive oil
- 1 onion, finely chopped
- 2 cloves garlic, minced
- 1 pound ground turkey
- 1 cup cooked quinoa
- 1 can (14.5 ounces) diced tomatoes, drained
- 1 teaspoon dried oregano
- 1 teaspoon dried basil
- Salt and pepper, to taste
- ½ cup shredded mozzarella cheese (optional)

Instructions:
1. Preheat the oven to 375 degrees F (190 degrees C).
2. Place the bell peppers in a baking dish, and set aside.
3. Heat the olive oil in a skillet over medium heat. Add the chopped onion and minced garlic, sautéing until the onion becomes translucent.
4. Add the ground turkey to the skillet, breaking it up as it cooks until it is no longer pink.
5. Stir in the cooked quinoa, diced tomatoes, oregano, and basil. Season with salt and pepper to taste. Cook together for another 5 minutes until everything is well combined.

6. Spoon the turkey and quinoa mixture into the hollowed-out bell peppers. Top with shredded mozzarella cheese if using.

7. Bake in the preheated oven for 25-30 minutes, or until the peppers are tender and the cheese is bubbly and golden.

Nutritional Information (per serving):

- Calories: 320
- Protein: 22g
- Carbohydrates: 27g
- Fat: 14g
- Fiber: 5g
- Sodium: 320mg

Serving Size: 1 stuffed pepper

Cooking Time: 45 minutes (20 minutes prep time, 25-30 minutes cooking time)

Grilled Vegetable and Hummus Flatbread

Ingredients:
- 1 whole wheat flatbread or naan
- 1/2 cup hummus
- 1 zucchini, sliced into thin rounds
- 1 bell pepper, any color, sliced
- 1 small red onion, sliced into rings
- 1 tablespoon olive oil
- Salt and pepper to taste
- 1/2 teaspoon dried herbs (such as thyme or oregano)
- Optional: a sprinkle of feta cheese or a drizzle of balsamic reduction

Instructions:
1. Preheat the grill to medium-high heat. Toss the sliced zucchini, bell pepper, and red onion with olive oil, salt, pepper, and dried herbs in a bowl.
2. Place the vegetables on the grill and cook for about 4-5 minutes per side or until they are nicely charred and tender.
3. While the vegetables are grilling, place the flatbread on the grill for about 1-2 minutes on each side, just long enough to get it warm and slightly crispy.
4. Spread the hummus evenly over the warm flatbread.

5. Arrange the grilled vegetables on top of the hummus. If desired, sprinkle with feta cheese or drizzle with balsamic reduction.

6. Cut into slices and serve warm.

Nutritional Information:

- Calories: 330 per serving
- Protein: 12 g
- Carbohydrates: 45 g
- Fat: 12 g
- Fiber: 8 g
- Sodium: 390 mg

Serving Size: 1 flatbread

Cooking Time: Preparation takes approximately 10 minutes, and cooking time is around 10 minutes, making for a total of 20 minutes from start to finish.

Broccoli and Cauliflower Cheese Bake

Ingredients:

- 1 head of broccoli, cut into florets
- 1 head of cauliflower, cut into florets
- 1 tablespoon of olive oil
- 1/2 teaspoon of salt
- 1/4 teaspoon of black pepper
- 1 cup of grated cheddar cheese
- 1/2 cup of milk
- 2 tablespoons of all-purpose flour
- 2 tablespoons of unsalted butter
- 1/2 teaspoon of mustard powder
- 1/4 teaspoon of garlic powder

Instructions:

1. Preheat the oven to 375°F (190°C).
2. Spread the broccoli and cauliflower florets on a baking sheet. Drizzle with olive oil and season with salt and pepper. Toss to coat evenly and roast in the oven for 15-20 minutes until they are just tender.
3. While the vegetables are roasting, prepare the cheese sauce. In a saucepan, melt the butter over medium heat. Stir in the flour to create a roux, cooking for about 1 minute until bubbly but not brown.

4. Gradually add the milk to the roux, whisking constantly to prevent lumps. Continue to cook and stir until the sauce thickens.
5. Remove the sauce from heat and stir in the grated cheese, mustard powder, and garlic powder until the cheese is melted and the sauce is smooth.
6. In a large baking dish, combine the roasted vegetables and cheese sauce, stirring to coat.
7. Bake in the preheated oven for 20-25 minutes, or until the top is bubbly and golden brown.

Nutritional Information:

- Calories: 250 per serving
- Protein: 12g
- Fat: 18g
- Carbohydrates: 15g
- Fiber: 4g
- Sodium: 300mg

Serving Size:

This recipe serves 4 people.

Cooking Time:

Total cooking time is approximately 60 minutes, which includes preparation, roasting, and baking.

Chapter: 4 Dinner Recipes

Grilled Chicken with Quinoa and Roasted Vegetables

Ingredients:

- 2 boneless, skinless chicken breasts
- 1 cup quinoa
- 2 cups water (for cooking quinoa)
- 1 zucchini, sliced
- 1 bell pepper, cut into 1-inch pieces
- 1 medium carrot, peeled and sliced
- 1 small red onion, cut into wedges
- 2 tablespoons olive oil
- 1 teaspoon dried thyme
- Salt and pepper to taste
- Fresh parsley, chopped (for garnish)

Instructions:

1. Preheat the grill to medium-high heat and preheat the oven to 400°F (200°C).
2. Rinse the quinoa under cold running water until the water runs clear. In a medium saucepan, bring 2 cups of water to a boil. Add quinoa, reduce heat to low, cover, and simmer for 15 minutes, or

until all water is absorbed. Remove from heat and let stand for 5 minutes, then fluff with a fork.

3. While the quinoa is cooking, toss zucchini, bell pepper, carrot, and red onion with olive oil, thyme, salt, and pepper. Spread the vegetables on a baking sheet and roast in the oven for about 20-25 minutes, or until tender and slightly caramelized.

4. Season the chicken breasts with salt and pepper. Grill for about 6-7 minutes per side, or until the internal temperature reaches 165°F (74°C) and the juices run clear.

5. To serve, spoon a base of fluffy quinoa onto each plate, top with grilled chicken, and arrange the roasted vegetables around the sides. Garnish with fresh parsley.

Nutritional Information (per serving):

- Calories: 450
- Protein: 35g
- Carbohydrates: 45g
- Fat: 15g
- Fiber: 6g
- Sodium: 200mg

Serving Size:

This recipe serves 2.

Cooking Time:

Preparation time is approximately 15 minutes, with an additional 30 minutes for cooking.

Baked White Fish with Garlic Spinach

Ingredients:

- 4 white fish fillets (such as cod or tilapia)
- 2 tablespoons olive oil
- 4 cloves garlic, minced
- 4 cups fresh spinach
- 1 lemon, juiced
- Salt and pepper, to taste
- Optional: fresh herbs such as parsley or dill for garnish

Instructions:

1. Preheat your oven to 375°F (190°C).
2. Line a baking sheet with foil and lightly grease it with a bit of olive oil.
3. Place the fish fillets on the baking sheet. Drizzle with half the olive oil and season with salt and pepper.
4. In a large skillet, heat the remaining olive oil over medium heat. Add garlic and sauté until fragrant, about 1 minute.
5. Add spinach to the skillet and sauté until it wilts, about 2-3 minutes. Squeeze half of the lemon juice over the spinach and stir to combine.
6. Spoon the garlic spinach mixture over the fish fillets.
7. Bake in the preheated oven for 12-15 minutes, or until the fish flakes easily with a fork.

8. Serve hot, garnished with fresh herbs if desired and the remaining lemon juice drizzled on top.

Nutritional Information (per serving):

- Calories: 210
- Protein: 23g
- Fat: 12g (2g saturated fat)
- Carbohydrates: 3g
- Fiber: 1g
- Sodium: 120mg

Serving Size:

- This recipe serves 4 individuals.

Cooking Time:

- Total preparation and cooking time is approximately 30 minutes.

Vegetable Lasagna with Ricotta Cheese

Ingredients:

- 1 zucchini, thinly sliced
- 1 yellow squash, thinly sliced
- 1 bell pepper (any color), julienned
- 1 small onion, thinly sliced
- 2 cups spinach, fresh
- 1 cup mushrooms, sliced
- 2 cloves garlic, minced
- 2 cups ricotta cheese
- 1 egg
- 2 tablespoons olive oil
- 2 cups marinara sauce
- 9 no-boil lasagna noodles
- 1 cup mozzarella cheese, shredded
- 1/4 cup Parmesan cheese, grated
- Salt and pepper to taste
- 1 teaspoon dried oregano
- 1 teaspoon dried basil

Instructions:

1. Preheat the oven to 375°F (190°C).
2. In a large skillet, heat olive oil over medium heat. Add garlic, zucchini, squash, bell pepper, onion, and mushrooms. Sauté until

vegetables are just tender, about 5-7 minutes. Stir in spinach and cook until wilted. Season with salt, pepper, oregano, and basil.
3. In a mixing bowl, combine ricotta cheese with an egg, blending until smooth.
4. Spread a thin layer of marinara sauce on the bottom of a 9x13 inch baking dish. Arrange 3 lasagna noodles over the sauce.
5. Layer half of the sautéed vegetables over the noodles, half of the ricotta mixture, and a third of the mozzarella cheese.
6. Repeat with another layer of noodles, remaining vegetables, ricotta mixture, and another third of the mozzarella cheese.
7. Top with the final layer of noodles, the remaining marinara sauce, the rest of the mozzarella, and sprinkle with Parmesan cheese.
8. Cover with foil and bake for 25 minutes. Remove foil and bake for another 10 minutes, or until the cheese is bubbly and golden.
9. Let stand for 10 minutes before slicing and serving.

Nutritional Information:

- Calories: 320 per serving
- Protein: 18g
- Carbohydrates: 35g
- Fat: 14g
- Sodium: 410mg
- Fiber: 3g

Serving Size:

- This recipe serves 8 people.

Cooking Time:
- Total preparation and cooking time is approximately 60 minutes, with an additional 10 minutes for cooling before serving.

Stuffed Bell Peppers with Ground Turkey and Herbs

For this recipe, the main ingredients include:

- 4 large bell peppers, tops cut, seeds removed
- 1 pound ground turkey
- 1 cup cooked quinoa
- 1 medium onion, finely chopped
- 2 cloves garlic, minced
- 1 cup spinach, chopped
- 1/4 cup fresh parsley, chopped
- 1 teaspoon dried oregano
- 1/2 teaspoon salt
- 1/4 teaspoon black pepper
- 1 tablespoon olive oil
- 1/2 cup low-sodium chicken broth
- 1/4 cup grated Parmesan cheese (optional)

Instructions:

1. Preheat the oven to 375°F (190°C).
2. In a skillet over medium heat, add the olive oil and sauté onion and garlic until translucent.
3. Add the ground turkey to the skillet, breaking it up as it cooks until browned and cooked through.

4. Stir in the cooked quinoa, spinach, parsley, oregano, salt, and pepper, and cook together for another 2-3 minutes until the spinach is wilted.
5. Stuff each bell pepper with the turkey and quinoa mixture, packing lightly until full.
6. Place the stuffed peppers upright in a baking dish and pour the chicken broth into the bottom of the dish.
7. Cover with foil and bake for 30 minutes. Remove the foil, top with grated Parmesan if using, and bake for another 10 minutes or until the peppers are tender and the cheese is melted.
8. Serve warm.

Nutritional Information:

Each serving (1 stuffed pepper) contains approximately:
- Calories: 290
- Protein: 26g
- Fat: 12g (with 3g saturated fat if using Parmesan)
- Carbohydrates: 23g
- Fiber: 5g
- Sodium: 320mg

Serving Size:

This recipe serves 4, with one stuffed pepper per serving.

Cooking Time:

Preparation time is about 15 minutes, and cooking time is 40 minutes, making a total time of 55 minutes.

Mushroom and Barley Soup

Ingredients:

- 1 tablespoon olive oil
- 1 onion, finely chopped
- 2 cloves garlic, minced
- 1 carrot, diced
- 1 celery stalk, diced
- 1 cup pearl barley, rinsed
- 8 ounces mushrooms, sliced (any variety)
- 6 cups low-sodium vegetable broth
- 2 teaspoons fresh thyme, chopped
- Salt and pepper to taste
- Parsley, chopped (for garnish)

Instructions:

1. Heat the olive oil in a large pot over medium heat. Add the chopped onion, garlic, carrot, and celery, and sauté until the vegetables are softened, about 5 minutes.
2. Add the sliced mushrooms to the pot and cook until they are browned and have released their juices, about 8 minutes.
3. Stir in the pearl barley and cook for another 2 minutes to lightly toast it, enhancing its nutty flavor.
4. Pour in the vegetable broth and bring the mixture to a boil. Reduce the heat to low, add the chopped thyme, and simmer covered for about 45 minutes, or until the barley is tender.

5. Season with salt and pepper to taste. Serve hot, garnished with chopped parsley.

Nutritional Information (per serving):

- Calories: 200
- Protein: 6g
- Carbohydrates: 44g
- Dietary Fiber: 9g
- Sugars: 4g
- Fat: 3g
- Sodium: 300mg

Serving Size: 1 cup
Cooking Time: Approximately 60 minutes

Beef Stew with Root Vegetables

Ingredients:

- 1 lb lean beef, cut into cubes
- 2 tablespoons olive oil
- 3 carrots, peeled and sliced
- 2 parsnips, peeled and sliced
- 1 large onion, chopped
- 2 cloves garlic, minced
- 2 potatoes, peeled and cubed
- 4 cups beef or vegetable broth, low sodium
- 1 teaspoon dried thyme
- Salt and pepper, to taste
- 2 tablespoons parsley, chopped (for garnish)

Instructions:

1. In a large pot, heat the olive oil over medium heat. Add the beef cubes and sear them until browned on all sides, about 5-7 minutes. Remove the beef and set aside.
2. In the same pot, add the onion and garlic, cooking until the onion becomes translucent.
3. Add the carrots, parsnips, and potatoes to the pot, stirring to mix.
4. Return the beef to the pot and add the broth. Stir in the thyme, salt, and pepper.

5. Bring the mixture to a boil, then reduce the heat and let it simmer, covered, for about 1 hour or until the vegetables and beef are tender.

6. Adjust seasoning to taste and garnish with chopped parsley before serving.

Nutritional Information (per serving):

- Calories: 330
- Protein: 26 g
- Carbohydrates: 30 g
- Fat: 12 g
- Fiber: 5 g
- Sodium: 300 mg

Serving Size: Serves 4

Cooking Time: Preparation time is about 20 minutes, with an additional 1 hour of cooking time.

Roasted Eggplant and Tomato Stew

Ingredients:

- 2 medium eggplants, peeled and cubed
- 3 large tomatoes, diced
- 1 onion, finely chopped
- 2 cloves garlic, minced
- 1 bell pepper, diced
- 2 tablespoons olive oil
- 1 teaspoon dried basil
- 1 teaspoon dried oregano
- Salt and pepper to taste
- 2 cups vegetable broth

Instructions:

1. Preheat the oven to 400 degrees Fahrenheit. Toss the cubed eggplant with one tablespoon of olive oil and spread it on a baking sheet. Roast in the oven for 25 minutes, turning once until the eggplant is tender and lightly browned.
2. While the eggplant is roasting, heat the remaining tablespoon of olive oil in a large pot over medium heat. Add the chopped onion and garlic, sautéing until the onion becomes translucent.
3. Add the bell pepper to the pot and cook for an additional 5 minutes until softened.
4. Stir in the roasted eggplant, diced tomatoes, vegetable broth, basil, oregano, salt, and pepper. Bring the mixture to a boil, then

reduce the heat and let it simmer for 20 minutes to allow the flavors to meld.

5. Taste and adjust the seasoning as needed before serving.

Nutritional Information:

- Calories: 200 per serving
- Protein: 3 g
- Fat: 10 g (mostly from olive oil, which provides healthy monounsaturated fats)
- Carbohydrates: 28 g
- Fiber: 9 g
- Sodium: 300 mg

Serving Size: Serves 4

Cooking Time: Prep time is about 15 minutes, cook time is 45 minutes, making the total time approximately 1 hour.

Cod in Parsley Sauce with Mashed Potatoes

Ingredients:

- 4 cod fillets (4-6 ounces each)
- 1 tablespoon olive oil
- Salt and pepper, to taste
- 2 cups milk
- 2 tablespoons unsalted butter
- 2 tablespoons flour
- 1/4 cup finely chopped fresh parsley
- 4 large potatoes, peeled and quartered
- 1/4 cup warm milk
- 2 tablespoons butter
- Salt, to taste

Instructions:

1. Begin by preparing the mashed potatoes. Boil the quartered potatoes in salted water until they are tender, about 20 minutes. Drain the water and mash the potatoes with warm milk and butter until smooth. Season with salt to taste and set aside, keeping them warm.
2. For the cod, heat olive oil in a skillet over medium heat. Season the cod fillets with salt and pepper, then place them in the skillet. Cook for about 4-5 minutes on each side or until the fish flakes

easily with a fork. Remove the cod from the skillet and keep warm.

3. In the same skillet, melt 2 tablespoons of butter. Whisk in the flour to create a roux, cooking for about 1 minute without browning. Gradually add 2 cups of milk, stirring continuously until the sauce thickens. Stir in the chopped parsley and season the sauce with salt and pepper to taste.

4. Serve the cooked cod fillets topped with the creamy parsley sauce and a side of mashed potatoes.

Nutritional Information:

- Calories: 450
- Protein: 38g
- Carbohydrates: 40g
- Fat: 18g
- Sodium: 190mg
- Fiber: 5g

Serving Size: Serves 4

Cooking Time: Preparation time is about 20 minutes, and cooking time is approximately 30 minutes, totaling about 50 minutes from start to finish.

Sweet Potato Shepherd's Pie

Ingredients:

- 2 large sweet potatoes, peeled and cubed
- 1 tablespoon olive oil
- 1 onion, finely chopped
- 2 carrots, peeled and diced
- 2 stalks of celery, diced
- 1 pound ground turkey or chicken
- 2 cloves garlic, minced
- 1 teaspoon dried thyme
- 1/2 teaspoon dried rosemary
- 1 tablespoon tomato paste
- 1 cup low-sodium chicken or vegetable broth
- 1 cup frozen peas
- Salt and pepper, to taste

Instructions:

1. Preheat the oven to 375°F (190°C).
2. Place the sweet potatoes in a large pot of boiling water and cook until tender, about 15-20 minutes. Drain and mash with a bit of salt and pepper; set aside.
3. While the potatoes are cooking, heat the olive oil in a large skillet over medium heat. Add the onion, carrots, and celery, and sauté until the vegetables are softened, about 5-7 minutes.

4. Add the ground turkey or chicken to the skillet and cook until browned, breaking it up as it cooks. Stir in the garlic, thyme, rosemary, and tomato paste, and cook for another 2 minutes.
5. Pour in the broth, bring to a simmer, and let the mixture cook down until slightly thickened, about 10 minutes. Stir in the frozen peas and season with salt and pepper.
6. Transfer the meat and vegetable mixture to a baking dish. Spread the mashed sweet potatoes over the top.
7. Bake in the preheated oven for 20-25 minutes, or until the topping is slightly golden.
8. Let the shepherd's pie cool for a few minutes before serving.

Nutritional Information:
- Serving size: 1/6 of the dish
- Calories: 250
- Protein: 18 g
- Fat: 8 g
- Carbohydrates: 28 g
- Fiber: 5 g
- Sugar: 8 g

Cooking Time:
- Prep time: 30 minutes
- Cook time: 45 minutes
- Total time: 75 minutes

Pasta with Pesto and Peas

Ingredients:

- 12 oz whole wheat pasta
- 1 cup fresh peas, or frozen and thawed
- 2 cups fresh basil leaves
- 2 cloves garlic, minced
- 1/4 cup pine nuts
- 1/2 cup grated Parmesan cheese
- 1/3 cup extra virgin olive oil
- Salt and pepper to taste
- Optional: 2 tbsp lemon juice for added flavor

Instructions:

1. Bring a large pot of salted water to a boil and cook the pasta according to the package instructions until al dente. In the last three minutes of cooking, add the peas to the boiling pasta.
2. While the pasta cooks, combine the basil, garlic, pine nuts, and Parmesan cheese in a food processor. Pulse until the ingredients are finely chopped.
3. With the processor running, slowly drizzle in the olive oil until the mixture forms a smooth paste. Season with salt and pepper, and add lemon juice if using.
4. Drain the pasta and peas, reserving a cup of the pasta water.

5. Return the pasta and peas to the pot and mix in the pesto sauce. Add reserved pasta water a little at a time to achieve a creamy consistency.

6. Serve warm, garnished with additional Parmesan if desired.

Nutritional Information (per serving):

- Calories: 450
- Protein: 16 g
- Fat: 22 g
- Carbohydrates: 52 g
- Fiber: 8 g
- Sodium: 190 mg

Serving Size:

- This recipe serves 4 people.

Cooking Time:

- Total preparation and cooking time is approximately 30 minutes.

Chapter: 5 Snacks and Sides

Healthy Snacking Options

Greek Yogurt with Berries and Honey

Ingredients:
- 1 cup plain Greek yogurt
- 1/2 cup fresh mixed berries (strawberries, blueberries, raspberries)
- 1 tablespoon honey
- 1 tablespoon chia seeds (optional)

Instructions:
1. Place the Greek yogurt in a bowl.
2. Top with mixed berries.
3. Drizzle honey over the berries.
4. Sprinkle chia seeds on top, if using.
5. Stir gently to combine or leave as is.

Nutritional Information (per serving):
- Calories: 200
- Protein: 15g
- Carbohydrates: 25g
- Fiber: 5g
- Sugars: 20g
- Fat: 5g

Serving Size: 1 bowl
Cooking Time: 5 minutes

Avocado and Cucumber Salad

Ingredients:
- 1 ripe avocado, diced
- 1 medium cucumber, sliced
- 1 tablespoon olive oil
- 1 tablespoon lemon juice
- Salt and pepper to taste
- 1 tablespoon chopped fresh dill (optional)

Instructions:
1. In a bowl, combine the diced avocado and cucumber slices.
2. Drizzle with olive oil and lemon juice.
3. Season with salt and pepper.
4. Toss gently to mix.
5. Sprinkle with fresh dill if desired.

Nutritional Information (per serving):
- Calories: 180
- Protein: 2g
- Carbohydrates: 10g
- Fiber: 7g

- Sugars: 2g
- Fat: 15g

Serving Size: 1 bowl
Cooking Time: 10 minutes

Baked Sweet Potato Fries

Ingredients:

- 2 large sweet potatoes, peeled and cut into fries
- 2 tablespoons olive oil
- 1 teaspoon paprika
- 1/2 teaspoon garlic powder
- 1/2 teaspoon salt
- 1/4 teaspoon black pepper

Instructions:

1. Preheat the oven to 425°F (220°C).
2. In a large bowl, toss the sweet potato fries with olive oil, paprika, garlic powder, salt, and pepper.
3. Spread the fries in a single layer on a baking sheet lined with parchment paper.
4. Bake for 25-30 minutes, turning halfway through, until the fries are crispy and golden.
5. Let cool slightly before serving.

Nutritional Information (per serving):

- Calories: 150
- Protein: 2g
- Carbohydrates: 25g
- Fiber: 4g
- Sugars: 5g
- Fat: 5g

Serving Size: 1 cup
Cooking Time: 30 minutes

Hummus and Veggie Sticks

Ingredients:

- 1 cup hummus (store-bought or homemade)
- 1 large carrot, cut into sticks
- 1 cucumber, cut into sticks
- 1 red bell pepper, cut into sticks
- 1 stalk celery, cut into sticks

Instructions:

1. Place the hummus in a serving bowl.
2. Arrange the carrot, cucumber, bell pepper, and celery sticks around the hummus.
3. Serve immediately or refrigerate until ready to eat.

Nutritional Information (per serving):
- Calories: 200
- Protein: 6g
- Carbohydrates: 22g
- Fiber: 8g
- Sugars: 7g
- Fat: 10g

Serving Size: 1 plate
Cooking Time: 10 minutes

Quinoa Salad with Lemon Vinaigrette

Ingredients:
- 1 cup cooked quinoa, cooled
- 1/2 cup cherry tomatoes, halved
- 1/4 cup diced red onion
- 1/4 cup chopped fresh parsley
- 2 tablespoons olive oil
- 1 tablespoon lemon juice
- Salt and pepper to taste

Instructions:
1. In a large bowl, combine the cooked quinoa, cherry tomatoes, red onion, and parsley.

2. In a small bowl, whisk together the olive oil, lemon juice, salt, and pepper.
3. Pour the vinaigrette over the quinoa salad and toss to combine.
4. Serve chilled or at room temperature.

Nutritional Information (per serving):
- Calories: 220
- Protein: 6g
- Carbohydrates: 30g
- Fiber: 5g
- Sugars: 3g
- Fat: 9g

Serving Size: 1 bowl
Cooking Time: 20 minutes (plus cooling time)

Recipes for Nutritious Sides

Sweet Potato and Quinoa Patties

Ingredients:
- 1 large sweet potato, peeled and cubed
- 1 cup cooked quinoa
- 1 small onion, finely chopped
- 1 garlic clove, minced
- 1/4 cup fresh parsley, chopped
- 1/2 teaspoon ground cumin
- 1/4 teaspoon ground turmeric
- Salt and pepper to taste
- 2 tablespoons olive oil

Instructions:
1. Steam the sweet potato until tender, then mash.
2. In a large bowl, combine the mashed sweet potato, cooked quinoa, onion, garlic, parsley, cumin, turmeric, salt, and pepper.
3. Form the mixture into small patties.
4. Heat olive oil in a large skillet over medium heat. Cook the patties for 3-4 minutes on each side until golden brown.
5. Serve warm.

Nutritional Information (per patty):
- Calories: 120
- Protein: 3g

- Carbohydrates: 18g
- Fat: 4g
- Fiber: 3g

Serving Size: 1 patty
Cooking Time: 30 minutes

Cucumber and Avocado Salad

Ingredients:
- 1 large cucumber, diced
- 1 ripe avocado, diced
- 1/4 cup red onion, finely chopped
- 1 tablespoon fresh lemon juice
- 2 tablespoons olive oil
- Salt and pepper to taste

Instructions:
1. In a large bowl, combine the cucumber, avocado, and red onion.
2. Drizzle with lemon juice and olive oil.
3. Season with salt and pepper, then toss gently to combine.
4. Serve immediately.

Nutritional Information (per serving):
- Calories: 160

- Protein: 2g
- Carbohydrates: 10g
- Fat: 14g
- Fiber: 7g

Serving Size: 1 cup
Cooking Time: 10 minutes

Baked Zucchini Fries

Ingredients:
- 2 medium zucchinis, cut into sticks
- 1/2 cup whole wheat breadcrumbs
- 1/4 cup grated Parmesan cheese
- 1/2 teaspoon garlic powder
- 1/2 teaspoon paprika
- Salt and pepper to taste
- 2 eggs, beaten

Instructions:
1. Preheat the oven to 425°F (220°C). Line a baking sheet with parchment paper.
2. In a bowl, mix breadcrumbs, Parmesan cheese, garlic powder, paprika, salt, and pepper.
3. Dip zucchini sticks into the beaten eggs, then coat with the breadcrumb mixture.

4. Arrange the zucchini sticks on the prepared baking sheet.

5. Bake for 20-25 minutes until golden and crispy.

6. Serve with a low-fat dip.

Nutritional Information (per serving):
- Calories: 100
- Protein: 5g
- Carbohydrates: 12g
- Fat: 4g
- Fiber: 2g

Serving Size: 1/2 cup
Cooking Time: 30 minutes

Greek Yogurt and Berry Parfait

Ingredients:
- 1 cup plain Greek yogurt
- 1/2 cup mixed berries (blueberries, strawberries, raspberries)
- 1 tablespoon honey
- 1/4 cup granola (optional)

Instructions:
1. In a serving glass, layer the Greek yogurt, berries, and honey.
2. If desired, top with granola for added crunch.
3. Serve immediately or chill in the refrigerator.

Nutritional Information (per serving):
- Calories: 180
- Protein: 10g
- Carbohydrates: 25g
- Fat: 4g
- Fiber: 3g

Serving Size: 1 cup
Cooking Time: 5 minutes

Hummus and Veggie Sticks

Ingredients:
- 1 can (15 oz) chickpeas, drained and rinsed
- 1/4 cup tahini
- 2 tablespoons olive oil
- 1 garlic clove
- Juice of 1 lemon
- 1/2 teaspoon ground cumin
- Salt to taste
- Assorted veggie sticks (carrots, celery, bell peppers)

Instructions:
1. In a food processor, combine chickpeas, tahini, olive oil, garlic, lemon juice, cumin, and salt. Blend until smooth.

2. Transfer the hummus to a serving bowl.
3. Serve with assorted veggie sticks.

Nutritional Information (per serving):
- Calories: 150
- Protein: 6g
- Carbohydrates: 18g
- Fat: 7g
- Fiber: 5g

Serving Size: 1/4 cup hummus with veggie sticks
Cooking Time: 10 minutes

Chapter: 6 Beverages and Smoothies

Juices and Smoothies to Support Hydration and Nutrition

Carrot and Ginger Juice

Ingredients:
- 4 large carrots
- 1 inch of fresh ginger root
- 1 apple
- 1/2 lemon, peeled

Instructions:
1. Wash all produce thoroughly.
2. Peel the ginger root and chop it roughly.
3. Core the apple and cut into wedges.
4. Run all ingredients through a juicer.
5. Stir the juice and serve immediately, or chill if preferred.

Nutritional Information:
Calories: 120, Carbs: 29g, Protein: 2g, Fat: 0.5g, Fiber: 6g

Serving Size:
Makes 2 servings.

Cooking Time:
Preparation time is about 10 minutes.

Kale and Pineapple Smoothie

Ingredients:
- 2 cups chopped kale, stems removed
- 1 cup frozen pineapple chunks
- 1 banana
- 1/2 cup plain Greek yogurt
- 1 cup water or coconut water

Instructions:
1. Place the kale, pineapple, banana, and Greek yogurt into a blender.
2. Add water or coconut water.
3. Blend on high until smooth.
4. Taste and adjust sweetness if necessary, adding a little honey if desired.

Nutritional Information:
Calories: 180, Carbs: 35g, Protein: 8g, Fat: 1g, Fiber: 3g

Serving Size:

Makes 2 servings.

Cooking Time:
Preparation time is about 5 minutes.

Watermelon Mint Juice

Ingredients:
- 2 cups chopped seedless watermelon
- 10 mint leaves
- 1/2 lime, peeled

Instructions:
1. Combine watermelon, mint leaves, and lime in a blender.
2. Blend until smooth.
3. Strain through a fine mesh sieve into glasses.

Nutritional Information:
Calories: 60, Carbs: 15g, Protein: 1g, Fat: 0g, Fiber: 1g

Serving Size:
Makes 2 servings.

Cooking Time:
Preparation time is about 8 minutes.

Avocado and Berry Smoothie

Ingredients:
- 1 ripe avocado, peeled and pitted
- 1/2 cup blueberries
- 1/2 cup strawberries
- 1 cup almond milk
- 1 tablespoon honey (optional)

Instructions:
1. Place all ingredients in a blender.
2. Blend on high until creamy and smooth.
3. Adjust sweetness with honey if needed.

Nutritional Information:
Calories: 220, Carbs: 27g, Protein: 3g, Fat: 12g, Fiber: 7g

Serving Size:
Makes 2 servings.

Cooking Time:
Preparation time is about 5 minutes.

Herbal Teas and Their Benefits

Green Ginger-Peach Smoothie

Ingredients:

- 1 ripe peach, sliced
- 1/2 cup fresh spinach
- 1 tablespoon grated fresh ginger
- 1 cup almond milk
- 1/2 banana

Instructions:

Combine all ingredients in a blender and blend until smooth. This smoothie is excellent for digestion due to the ginger, and the peach adds natural sweetness.
Nutritional Information (per serving):
Calories: 150, Protein: 3g, Carbohydrates: 35g, Fat: 1.5g
Serving Size: 1 serving
Preparation Time: 5 minutes

Hydrating Cucumber-Mint Water

Ingredients:

- 1 cucumber, thinly sliced
- 10 fresh mint leaves
- 2 quarts of water

Instructions:

Place the cucumber and mint leaves in a large pitcher. Add water and refrigerate for at least 1 hour to allow the flavors to infuse.

Nutritional Information (per serving):
Calories: 0, Protein: 0g, Carbohydrates: 0g, Fat: 0g
Serving Size: 1 cup
Preparation Time: 5 minutes (plus infusing time)

Soothing Ginger Tea

Ingredients:
- 1 inch of fresh ginger root, thinly sliced
- 2 cups of water
- Honey or lemon to taste (optional)

Instructions:
Boil water and add sliced ginger. Simmer for 10-15 minutes. Strain and add honey or lemon if desired. Ginger is known for its anti-inflammatory properties and can help soothe digestive issues.

Nutritional Information (per serving):
Calories: varies if honey or lemon is added
Serving Size: 1 cup
Preparation Time: 20 minutes

Berry Almond Milk Smoothie

Ingredients:

- 1/2 cup blueberries
- 1/2 cup raspberries
- 1 cup almond milk
- 1 tablespoon flax seeds

Instructions:
Blend all ingredients until smooth. This smoothie is rich in antioxidants from the berries and omega-3 fatty acids from the flax seeds.
Nutritional Information (per serving):
Calories: 200, Protein: 3g, Carbohydrates: 28g, Fat: 9g
Serving Size: 1 serving
Preparation Time: 5 minutes

Herbal Chamomile Tea

Ingredients:
- 2 tablespoons dried chamomile flowers
- 1 cup boiling water

Instructions:
Steep chamomile flowers in boiling water for 5-7 minutes. Strain and serve. Chamomile can help reduce inflammation and aid in sleep.

Nutritional Information (per serving):
Calories: 2, Protein: 0g, Carbohydrates: 0.5g, Fat: 0g

Serving Size: 1 cup
Preparation Time: 10 minutes

Chapter: 7 Tips for Eating Well During Treatment

Managing Common Digestive Issues

Managing common digestive issues is crucial for individuals undergoing treatment for pancreatic cancer, as these complications can significantly impact quality of life and nutritional intake. Digestive problems such as nausea, vomiting, diarrhea, and constipation are frequent side effects of both the disease and its treatment. Addressing these symptoms effectively can help maintain an optimal nutritional status, which is vital for recovery and overall well-being.

Nausea is one of the most common issues faced by pancreatic cancer patients. To combat this, it is recommended to eat small, frequent meals throughout the day instead of three large ones. Keeping the stomach slightly filled can prevent it from becoming upset, which is often a precursor to nausea. Cold or room-temperature foods are also advised since they have less aroma, which can sometimes trigger nausea. Ginger tea or ginger supplements are beneficial as well, as ginger is known to have natural anti-nausea properties.

For those experiencing vomiting, it is important to focus on hydration. Losing too many fluids and electrolytes can lead to dehydration, worsening the patient's condition. Oral rehydration solutions or electrolyte-rich drinks should be consumed to replenish lost fluids and maintain electrolyte balance. Once vomiting subsides, reintroducing solid foods slowly with bland, easy-to-digest options such as toast, rice, or bananas is essential.

Diarrhea can lead to significant fluid and nutrient losses. Foods rich in soluble fiber, like oatmeal, applesauce, and bananas, can help solidify stools and slow down bowel movements. Avoiding high-fat, greasy, or very sweet foods is crucial as these can exacerbate symptoms. Probiotics, found in yogurt or in supplement form, can also help restore the natural balance of the gut flora, aiding in digestion and stool formation.

Constipation, on the other hand, is best managed by increasing fiber intake through foods such as vegetables, fruits, whole grains, and legumes. Adequate fluid intake is equally important, as water helps fiber function more effectively. Regular, mild physical activity can also stimulate bowel movements. However, it's important for patients to speak with their healthcare provider before starting any new exercise regimen.

Addressing enzyme insufficiency is another critical aspect of managing digestive issues in pancreatic cancer patients. The pancreas may not produce enough enzymes to break down food, leading to malabsorption and weight loss. Pancreatic enzyme replacement therapy (PERT) is often prescribed to aid digestion. These enzymes should be taken with every meal and snack to ensure proper food breakdown and nutrient absorption.

Lastly, creating a comfortable eating environment can also alleviate some digestive symptoms. Eating in a relaxed setting, taking time to eat slowly, and thoroughly chewing food can all help improve digestion. Emotional support from friends and family during meals can also positively affect digestion and appetite. Engaging in light conversation or listening to soothing music during meals can make eating a more pleasant and effective experience, contributing to better digestive health and overall wellness.

Meal Planning and Preparation Tips

Effective meal planning and preparation are crucial for pancreatic cancer patients to maintain their nutrition during treatment. It is important to create a meal plan that accommodates the fluctuating energy levels and varying appetite that patients often experience. Setting up a weekly meal plan can help ensure that nutritious meals are available when needed, without requiring daily cooking. By planning ahead, patients and caregivers can manage energy better and make sure that eating well remains a priority even on difficult days.

To facilitate easier meal preparation, it is recommended to prepare ingredients in advance. Washing and chopping vegetables, marinating proteins, and portioning out servings can make assembling meals much quicker and simpler. This approach is especially beneficial on days following treatment, when fatigue might be more pronounced. Ready-to-cook ingredients help in putting together nutritious meals in less time, which is less daunting for both the patient and their caregiver.

Freezing meals is another effective strategy that can help patients receive adequate nutrition with minimal effort. Cooking large batches of stews, casseroles, or soups and freezing them in single-serving containers can provide quick, easy meals that only require reheating. This not only saves time but also ensures that the patient has access to homemade, healthful food on days they feel too tired or unwell to cook.

It's also useful to focus on energy-dense foods that provide more calories, proteins, and nutrients in smaller volumes. Meals enriched with healthy fats like avocado, olive oil, or nuts can offer the needed energy without the bulk of larger meals, which might be off-putting when appetite is reduced. Smoothies are a great option for incorporating nutritious calories and can be easily tailored to personal taste and nutritional needs.

Another important aspect is the flexibility in meal timing and frequency. Traditional meal schedules might not work for someone undergoing cancer treatment. Instead, eating smaller, more frequent meals or snacks can be more manageable and less overwhelming. This also ensures a steady intake of calories and nutrients throughout the day, which is vital for maintaining energy levels and managing weight.

Creating a comfortable and inviting eating environment can also significantly enhance the eating experience. A pleasant setting, perhaps with soothing music or a nice view, can help make mealtime more enjoyable and less stressful. Encouraging the social aspect of dining by eating with family or friends when possible can also provide emotional support and stimulate appetite.

Lastly, communication with healthcare providers about the diet is essential. They can offer guidance tailored to the specific side effects and nutritional needs of the patient. Dietitians specializing in oncology can provide valuable insights into how to adapt diet plans as treatment progresses and needs change. Regular updates and consultations ensure that the dietary approach remains effective and appropriate for the patient's current health status.

conclusion

Concluding the journey through the "Pancreatic Cancer Diet Cookbook for Beginners," it becomes evident that this guide is more than just a collection of recipes—it's a crucial tool designed to empower those affected by pancreatic cancer. Through its carefully curated meals and in-depth guidance, this cookbook addresses the specific nutritional challenges posed by the disease and its treatments, providing practical solutions that can help enhance the quality of life for patients.

This cookbook aims to make nutritional management accessible and less daunting. By breaking down the complexities of dietary needs during such a challenging time, it gives patients and their caregivers the confidence to prepare meals that not only nourish but also comfort and heal. It recognizes the power of food in the healing process, not just as sustenance but as a crucial component of the treatment regimen.

The diverse array of recipes ensures that there is something suitable for different tastes and dietary tolerances, accommodating common side effects like nausea, decreased appetite, and taste changes. This adaptability is key to maintaining an adequate nutritional intake, crucial for sustaining the body's strength and resilience during therapy.

Furthermore, the book's emphasis on hydration, meal planning, and the psychological impact of sharing meals highlights the holistic approach needed when dealing with pancreatic cancer. It is not only the body that needs care and nourishment but also the spirit. Creating enjoyable meal experiences can provide emotional boosts and foster connections with loved ones, essential during times of illness.

The inclusion of sections on hydration and snacks, along with preparation tips, enables patients and their families to integrate these dietary strategies into their daily routines seamlessly. These elements ensure that the diet remains balanced, practical, and responsive to the evolving needs of the patient.

Importantly, the "Pancreatic Cancer Diet Cookbook for Beginners" also serves as a bridge to the medical care team, offering a basis for discussions about nutrition and its role in cancer care. It supports the collaborative effort between patients, caregivers, and healthcare providers to tailor dietary approaches to individual needs.

In conclusion, this cookbook does more than feed the body; it nurtures the soul and fortifies the spirit. It stands as a testament to the importance of diet in cancer care and a reminder of the profound impact thoughtful, well-prepared meals can have on the well-being of those facing pancreatic cancer. By embracing the guidance within these pages, patients and caregivers can face the road ahead with more confidence, equipped with the tools to manage one of the most critical aspects of cancer treatment: nutrition.

www.ingramcontent.com/pod-product-compliance
Lightning Source LLC
Chambersburg PA
CBHW050110230526
45470CB00004B/1757